Frankie's FOIBLES

A story about a boy who worries

Kath Grimshaw

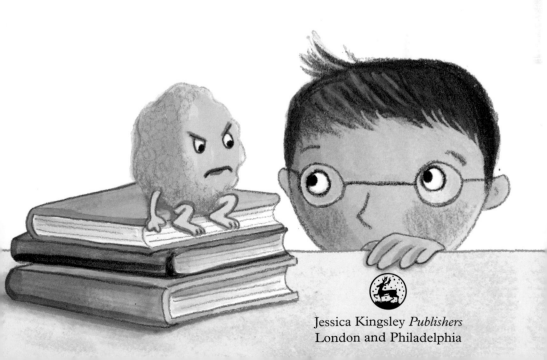

Jessica Kingsley *Publishers*
London and Philadelphia

First published in 2016
by Jessica Kingsley Publishers
73 Collier Street
London N1 9BE, UK
and
400 Market Street, Suite 400
Philadelphia, PA 19106, USA

www.jkp.com

Library of Congress Cataloging in Publication Data
A CIP catalog record for this book is available from the Library of Congress

British Library Cataloguing in Publication Data
A CIP catalogue record for this book is available from the British Library

ISBN 978 1 84905 695 3
eISBN 978 1 78450 210 2

Printed and bound in China

For Sam and Laurie

And many thanks to my friend and editorial whizz
Katharine Walkden.

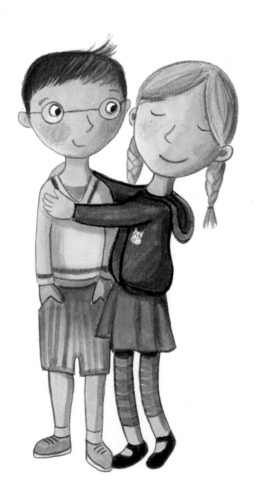

Frankie is feeling glum. He has just moved to Plum Street with his mum.

"We're starting fresh," she says, with a smile.

Frankie is happy that their new house is around the corner from Granny. But he's worried as well. Tomorrow he's starting a new school, filled with children he doesn't know.

He knows the way there (left down Plum Street, right up Leonard Lane, then left down Radish Road), but he thinks he might get lost at school. If only he had a map to memorize, with corridors, classrooms, cupboards and corners to hide in.

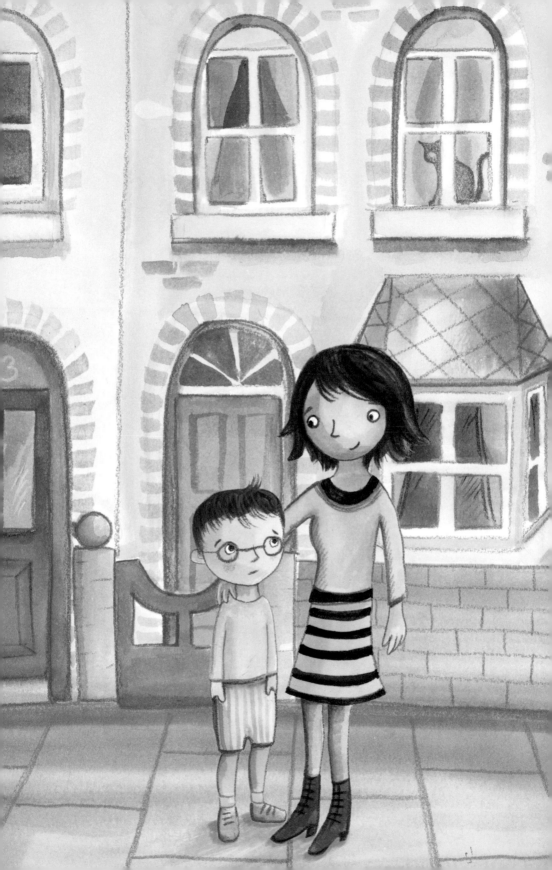

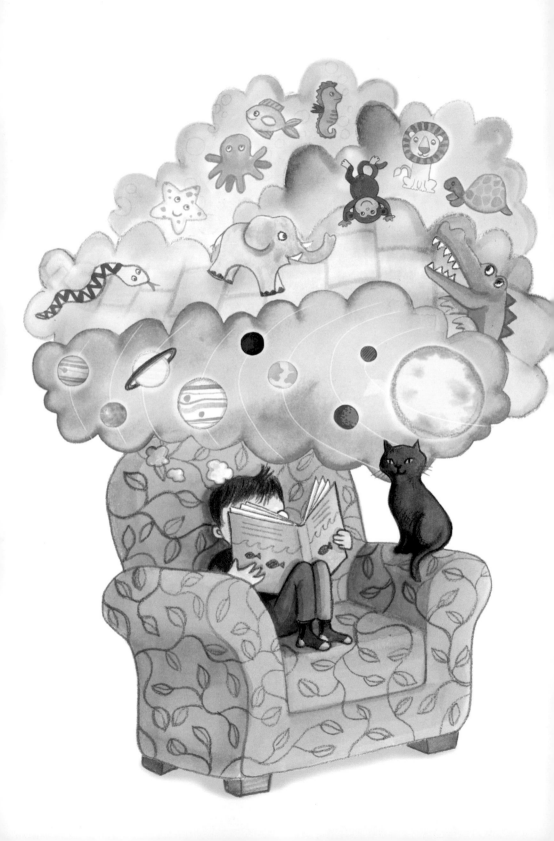

Frankie is really good at remembering things. Stuff he reads in books, like how far all the planets are from the sun and all the animals in his encyclopedia.

And stuff he's worked out by himself, like how many days he has lived on the earth (2,348) and how many paving stones there are on the way to his new school (587).

He's really *not* good at making new friends. Quite often he just doesn't know what to say. Sometimes, strange things scare him and weird things worry him. Like what might happen if he steps on a crack in the pavement. Five hundred and eighty seven paving stones – that's a lot of cracks.

On Monday morning Frankie brushes his teeth for three minutes. Mum says that two minutes is long enough, but three is his favourite number. Actually, he likes everything to be three. And he wants to be extra sure that bacteria aren't going to eat holes in his teeth.

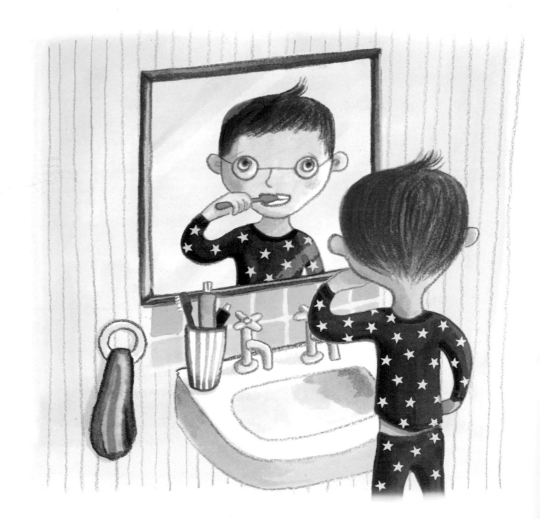

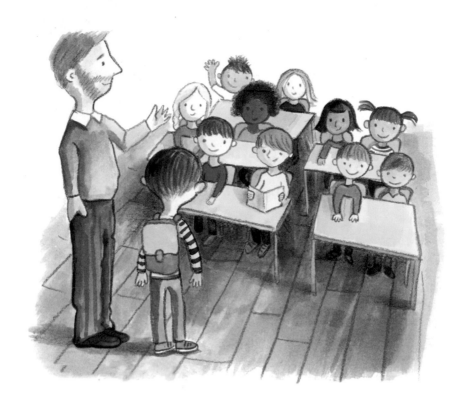

At his new school the children all smile at him. But he's too scared to smile back. So he doesn't talk to anyone, just in case.

For lunch he eats three sandwiches, three pieces of cucumber and three strawberries. There's a note in his lunch box, from his mum. It says, *Remember to smile, I love you.* Frankie tries curling up the corners of his mouth, but the boys on the next table laugh, so he curls them down again.

After school, he walks to Granny's house. Granny has bad knees so he walks by himself. That's okay, because he remembers the way.

On the corner of Leonard Lane, three big boys are waiting with their hands on their hips. They watch him step carefully over the cracks in the pavement. Butterflies flutter in his tummy.

"Excuse me," he says, in a tiny voice. "Can I get past?" He feels like he is shrinking as they stick out their chests and blow up like puffer fish.

Frankie wants to run away, he really does. But he might step on the cracks. He is shipwrecked on his paving stone.

If only he could fly.

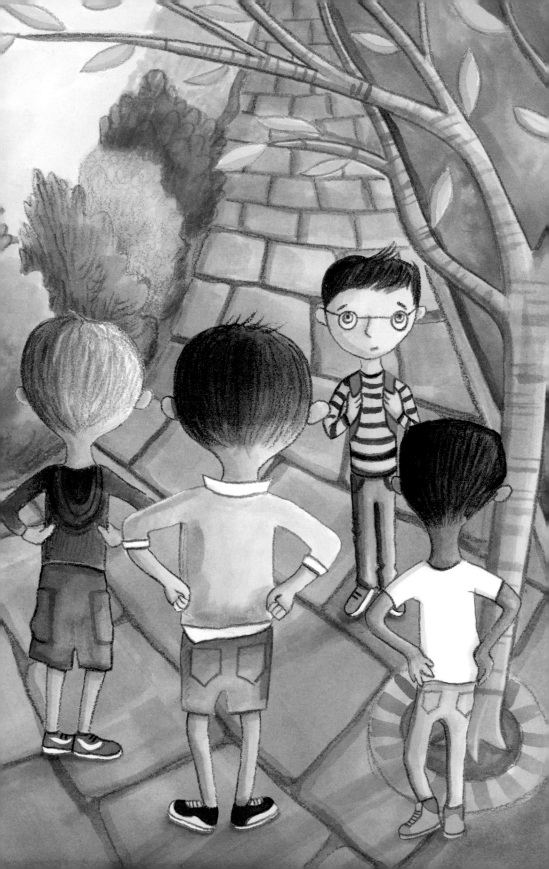

The boys are mean. They push him into the hedge, and shake his bag until pens, books and lunch box clatter and scatter all over the pavement. They laugh, and run away, their feet thundering down the street.

Frankie picks up his pencils. One has rolled right into a crack. His new homework book has landed in a puddle.

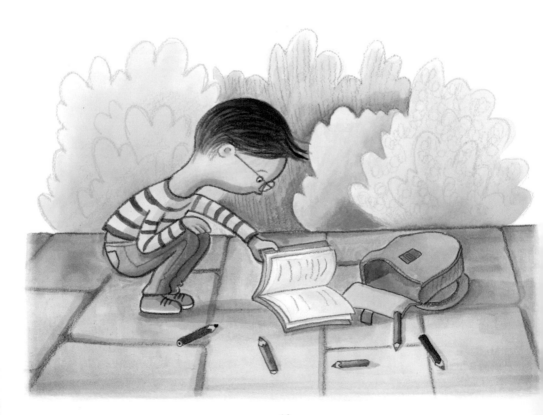

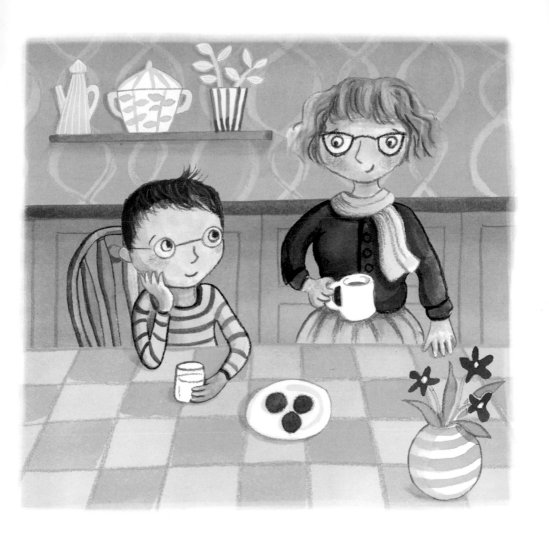

A little later he sits at Granny's table with three chocolate chip cookies and a glass of milk.

"What's wrong my darling?" she asks. "You seem sad."

He practises his fake smile and says, "Nothing Granny." He thinks he got away with it.

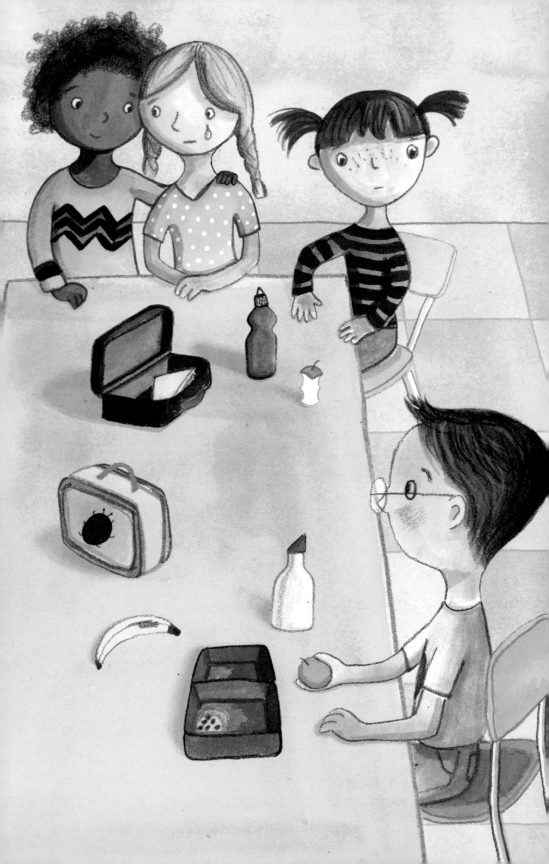

Frankie sits by himself at lunchtime again. At the other end of the table a girl with yellow pigtails is crying. Big wet tears plop onto her sandwich.

"What's wrong?" asks Frankie.

The crying girl sniffs. Her eyes and nose are red. She says, sadly, "My grandma gave me a cat brooch for my birthday. I lost it on the way to school. I'm never going to see it again." And then she starts to cry again.

"Her grandma died last year," whispers her friend.

Frankie doesn't know what to say. A brand new worry blooms in his chest.

Uh, oh. The big boys are waiting again. As Frankie turns the corner and sees them, his tummy twists upside down. He is marooned on his paving stone. The boys push him over and empty his bag again.

When he gets back to Granny's, she sees the tears on his cheeks. She opens her arms wide and folds him into a special big Granny bear hug. "Why don't you tell me what's making you sad?" she says.

Granny makes him a cup of hot chocolate with a mountain of mini-marshmallows. He takes a deep breath and tells her about the big boys, and how he can't run away. How he's scared of them, but that he's even more scared of what might happen if he steps on the cracks.

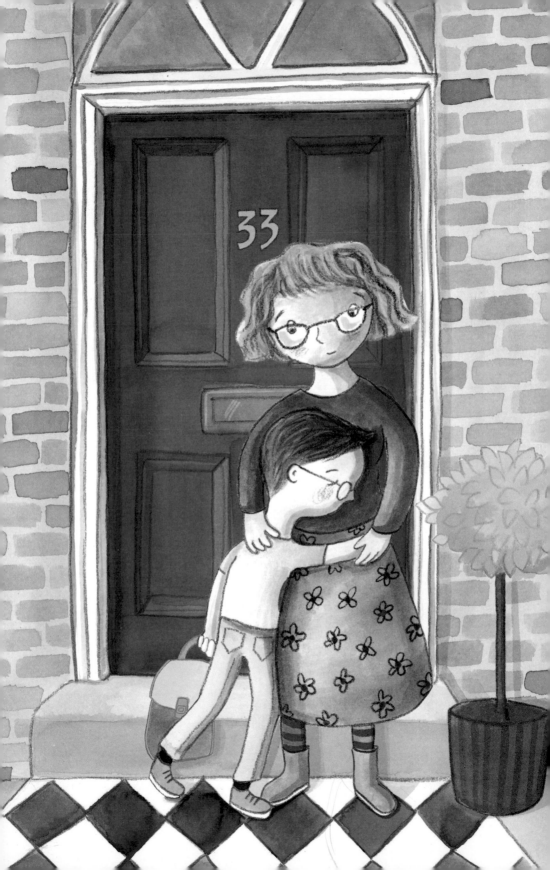

Granny has a think about this. "Well, Frankie, quite apart from those bully boys, who we will have to deal with, I think you might have got yourself some pesky foibles."

"What are foibles?" he asks.

"I'm not really sure where they come from, but what they *do* is whisper worries in your ear and tell you mean or silly thoughts that make you feel scared or sad. The more you try to tell them to go away, the more they keep popping back. They are horrid little bullies, just like those boys."

Frankie feels a warm glow growing inside him. It might be the hot chocolate or it might be because Granny seems to know exactly how he's feeling. "Do you have foibles too Granny?" he asks.

"Yes, my love. I have a tricky, sticky one who makes me think I haven't shut the front door. I have to walk all the way home to check again, with my poor knees!"

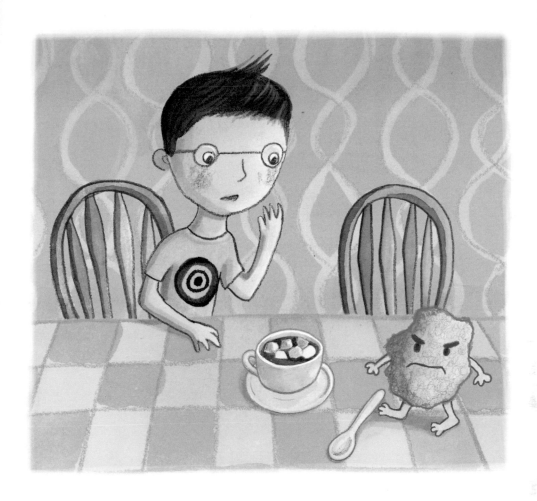

Just then, Frankie notices a funny creature on the table. It looks a bit like a potato, with skinny arms and legs and a cross, green face. Frankie blinks and rubs his eyes but the thing is still there, trying to kick a teaspoon with its grumpy feet.

It must be a foible!

"But what can we do about them Granny? How do we make them go away?" The foible pokes out its tongue. Granny hasn't noticed it.

"The only thing to do is to try your best to ignore them, Frankie, just like those bullies. It's not always easy, but we will all help you as best we can."

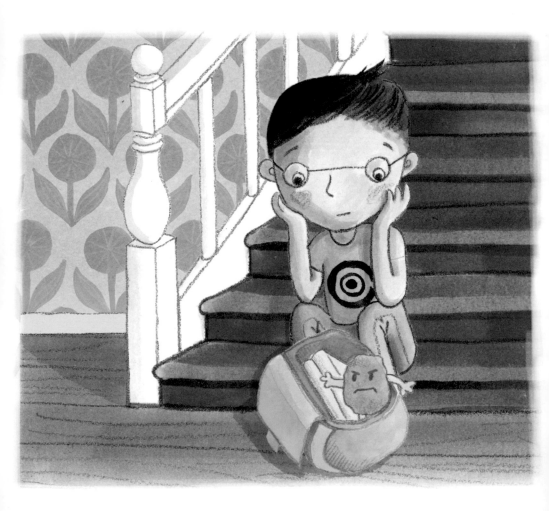

When Mum comes to pick him up, she and Granny chat in the kitchen for ages. Frankie sits on the stairs and looks at the foible sitting in his bag. Now he can see it, he doesn't know how to make it go away. It whispers, *"You still need to keep your eyes on that pavement. Don't step on the cracks, or who knows what might happen..."*

Next morning he feels brave and asks Mum for four sandwiches instead of three. But now there are two foibles in his school bag. The new one has a blue lumpy face and eyes like raisins. It sniggers at him, *"Four sandwiches? What are you thinking? You need to have three! And I hope you brushed your teeth for three minutes. Who knows what bad things might happen?"*

He takes a deep breath and buckles up his bag, trying to ignore the muffled mumbles from inside.

On the way to school, one of the foibles climbs out of Frankie's backpack. It cackles in his ear as Frankie steps carefully over each crack in the pavement, *"Look what happens when you try to forget about me. You can't get rid of me that easily!"*

He thinks about what Granny said – that it's not always easy. For a little while he had felt better and braver, learning about the foibles. But they are still here, annoying him, and he feels cross and cranky.

So, as he walks, he keeps his eyes glued to the ground, stepping carefully over the dark gaps. Then, something glints at him from the shadow of a pavement crack. The slab is broken with a missing corner and spiky grass growing from it. He picks up a shiny object hiding in the grass – it is a silver cat with a pin in the back.

He remembers the girl with the yellow pigtails.

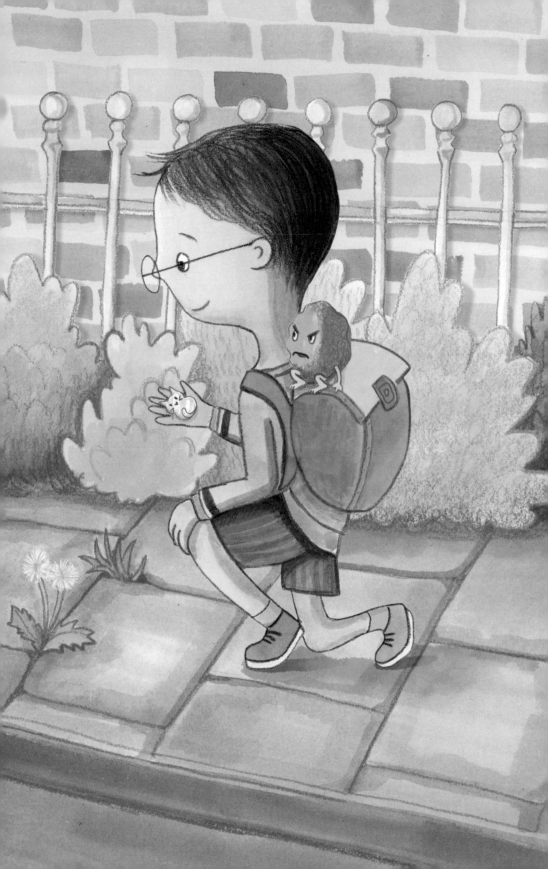

In the lunch hall, the girl and her friends are sitting together. Frankie takes a deep breath and asks, "Do you mind if I sit here?"

The foibles wriggle in his bag, but the girl with the yellow pigtails smiles at him. This makes him brave. He says, "I think I found your brooch on the way to school," and unfolds his hand. In his palm, the silver cat winks up at them.

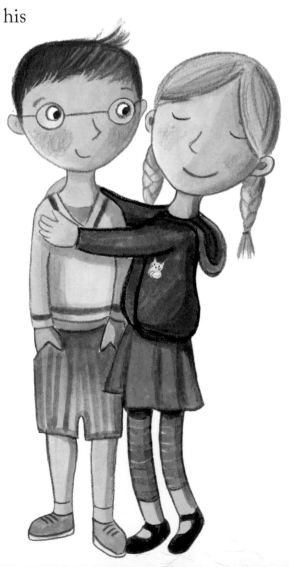

The girls all squeal at once, and Frankie's ears go *ping!* The girl with the yellow pigtails leaps up out of her chair and hugs him tightly, until his face feels hot and pink.

"Where did you find it?" she asks, pinning it to her top.

"On Radish Road, on my way to school," he says. "It was stuck in a crack in the pavement."

"Oh, thank you soooo much," says the girl. "My name is Milly, what's yours?"

Frankie's foibles are quiet as he chats to Milly and her friends. She lives on Leonard Lane too. "We could walk home from school together!" Milly suggests.

"That would be great!" says Frankie, and he smiles. But he's not smiling as he waits for Milly at the school gate. And the foibles are noisy. They are whispering to him.

"What if the big boys are there again?"

"What if they scare Milly too?"

"What if she laughs?"

Perhaps he should just walk home on his own?

But Milly is here now. She sees his worried face and asks, "What's wrong Frankie?"

He doesn't know what to say. Then he remembers how much better he felt when he told Granny about his foibles. So, as they walk along, he tells Milly all about it too: the cracks in the pavement, the bullies, the foibles.

"Oh, it sounds a bit like when I go somewhere high up – I'm always scared that I'll fall over the edge, even when I know I'm safe."

"I didn't think anyone else had bad thoughts," says Frankie. "I just thought I was weird."

"A thought is just a thought, silly," she says, firmly. "You have to do bad things to be bad."

Frankie looks ahead of them to the end of the road, "Speaking of bad people..." he says. There they are. The three bullies, standing on the corner.

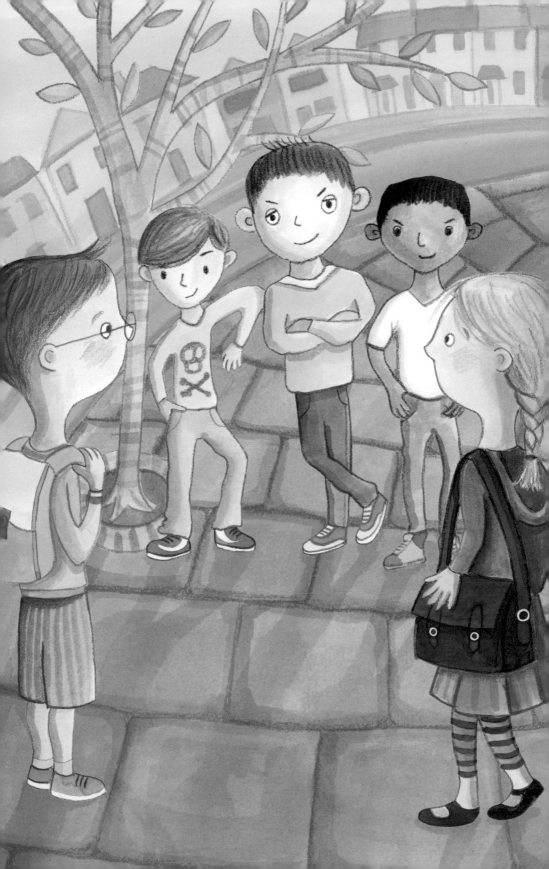

"Oooh, Frankie's got a girlfriend..." says one of the boys.

Frankie's cheeks turn pink. He can hear his foibles tutting and wriggling and giggling in his backpack.

"Does your girlfriend know you can't step on the ickle wickle cwacks, Frankie?" grins another boy. "Look, Frankie's stuck in the mud..."

Milly whispers in Frankie's ear, "Let's run for it!"

"But the cracks!" squeal his foibles.

"You can do it. Ignore them." Milly grabs his hand, and they start to run.

The bullies aren't expecting this. The children crash through them and up the path. Frankie's backpack is as light as a feather. His feet hardly touch the ground. He feels as though he is flying.

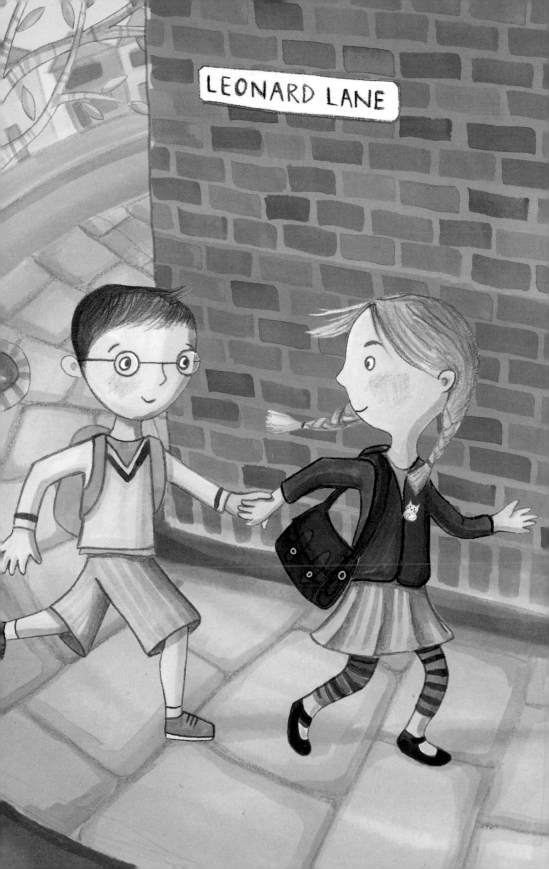

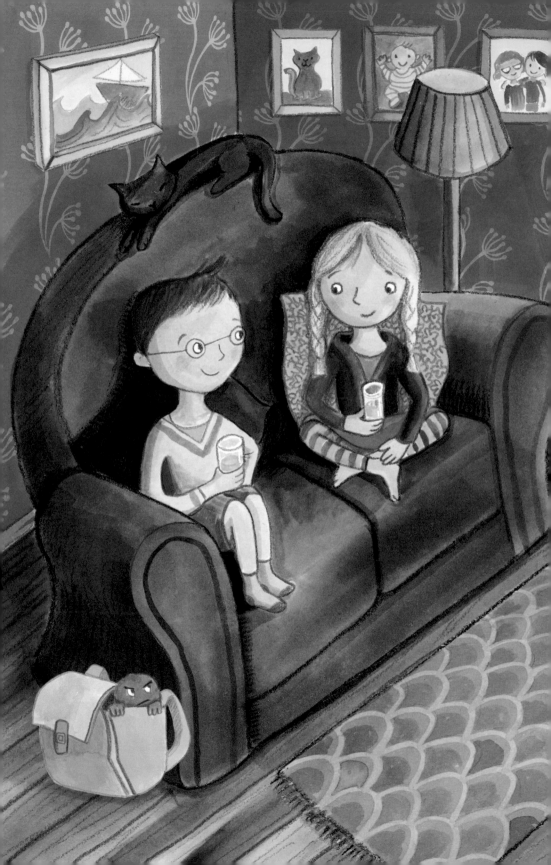

One of the foibles has gone. A moment ago Frankie sneaked a peek in his backpack and there's no sign of old grumpy green-face. Lumpy blue is still in there, grumbling at being left on his own. But suddenly Frankie knows that he might not be stuck with him forever. He stepped on the cracks and nothing bad happened.

In fact, something very good has happened. He's made a new friend, and right now they are sitting on Granny's sofa, drinking apple juice. Granny and Milly's mum are having a cup of tea.

"Do you know, Frankie's the fastest runner I've ever seen!" says Milly.

Frankie has a proper grin on his face. A big one that stretches from ear to ear. He can't wait to tell his mum.